I Am Hip Hop, I Am Health

I0101553

I Am Hip Hop, I Am Health

Dr. Ross Flowers, Dr. Gary Davis,
Dr. Che Joplin

Cover Art
By
J Graphix
(502) 649-1152

‹♦›

Copyright © 2007
Dr. Ross Flowers, Dr. Gary Davis, & Dr. Che Joplin
All Rights Reserved
All rights reserved. No part of this book
may be reproduced in any form, except for the inclusion of quotations in a review,
without permission in writing from the authors or publisher.

‹♦›

I Am Hip-Hop, I Am Health® / Dr. Ross Flowers, Dr. Gary Davis, & Dr. Che Joplin /
1st Edition
ISBN-1: 978-1-4243-3741-5 (pbk)
First paperback edition published in 2007 by the authors
I Am Hip-Hop, I Am Health is a registered trademark of Dr. Ross Flowers, Dr. Gary
Davis, & Dr. Che Joplin

‹♦›

All rights reserved. No part of this book may be reproduced in any form, except for
the inclusion of quotations in a review, without permission in writing from the authors
or publisher.

Copyright © 2007 Dr. Ross Flowers, Dr. Gary Davis, Dr. Che Joplin
All rights reserved.
ISBN: 1-4243-3741-0
ISBN-13: 9781-424337415

Visit www.booksurge.com to order additional copies.

I Am Hip Hop, I Am Health

Track List

Push Play

You are about to embark on a transformational journey toward hip-hop and how it can affect health for the better. I Am Hip-Hop, I Am Health is an identity embodied in an appreciation and commitment to the hip-hop culture and to healthy living. It doesn't matter what age you are, what the condition of your body and mind is, or how long you have or have not been on the path to seeking health and wellness, if you want to change your lifestyle, this book is for you.

The information given here will help you to alter your belief system and take charge of your health. The, I Am Hip-Hop, I Am Health, movement was created to address six deadly health disparities that are plaguing American hip-hop communities. They are: Obesity, Cardiovascular disease, Diabetes, Hypertension, Cancer and HIV/AIDS.

This book was written by three, young, hip healthcare professionals with several goals: 1) merge the hip-hop community with the health care community in order to increase the awareness of chronic conditions that are associated with morbidity and mortality; 2) educate young, hip-hop communities about health disparities and improved health practices; and 3) educate the reader about the risks and damaging effects of uncontrolled diseases.

I have been a healthcare provider for more than 10 years and I believe that we should all experience quality and quantity of life. It is difficult to balance the forces of life, especially stress, disease, disappointments and neglect. But too often, we ignore health issues to accommodate the stressors of daily life not realizing that what we ignore does not go away. The ideas and concepts of this book are written to nourish and strengthen the minds and bodies of those living behind and through the music.

This book embraces hip-hop as a musical genre that has built a bridge between the young and the old. It does so to help build a relationship that moves beyond music. The principles explained in this book recognize no color, race or cultural differences. Their purpose is to create a new you and place you on the path of health and wellness with an ounce of hip-hop. Keep a journal, study and read the principles as often as you need until you reach your goals. And remember, "Better Health through Better Living" is the goal that we all must strive to accomplish.

Michelle L. Fuselier, MD

Fast-Forward

It has been more than thirty years and hip-hop has evolved into a global cultural phenomenon. It is music, but it is more than music. Hip-hop is poetry, dance, art, rap, music, graffiti, videos, fashion, and technology. Hip-hop is organic. It is alive. Hip-hop is the cognitive expression of youth throughout the world. Hip-hop is youth consciousness and lifestyle.

Hip-hop is also interdisciplinary. The health of people and communities in America and throughout the world is one of the greatest interests to the hip-hop generation. The fastest growing demographic in the human population are children and young adults. Yet when it comes to individual and public health issues and conditions, hip-hop more than any other cultural phenomena is not only where the higher aspirations of youth are expressed, it is also the means by which the presence or absence of good health is articulated with the passionate force of youth who cry out for a better quality of life.

Good health and wellness does not happen by osmosis. You have to work at being healthy. The genius of I AM HIP-HOP— I AM HEALTH is that this book is one of the first publications that affirms the positive attributes of hip-hop culture as a means by which vital health and wellness issues, concerns, programs, public policy and education will effectively be transmitted to hundreds of millions of youth throughout the world.

Hip-hop is no longer just an American art form or cultural expression; hip-hop is all over the world and growing stronger and stronger everyday. Even the United Nations is now exploring ways and means to utilize hip-hop to enhance the communication of vital and important information to youth internationally.

Dr. Ross Flowers, Dr. Gary Davis and Dr. Che Joplin in I AM HIP-HOP—I AM HEALTH have made an important contribution to pubic health education and awareness. This book also captures the spirit of hip-hop. Promoting awareness among young people about the rewards of knowledge and living life where wellness is at the core of youth consciousness, attitude and actions is of the utmost importance.

It is said that having information and knowledge is power. That is true. Yet for the majority of the world's population being able to take preventative and corrective actions with respect to health issues is a matter of life and death. Young people all over the world are crying out for a better quality of life. Each successive generation should be able to experience a better quality of health care than the previous generation. It is unfortunate that the reality for millions of youth in America and throughout the international community is that poverty and poor health care are both on the rise. With all the advances in science and technology, the United Nations and the international community will have to do better to transform the lives of hundreds of millions of young people who want to get out of poverty and to enjoy the benefits of good health and wellness. This is not an impossible goal. This is not an impossible dream.

Hip-hop was born in America among African Americans and Latino Americans over thirty years ago. Today in every nation and on every continent hip-hop music and cultural expressions have grasped the heart and soul of youth. Hip-hop has evolved to transcend race and the ideological divisions of the past. I am encouraging all of the talented and gifted hip-hop artists of today across the world to take the contents of this book seriously. We need "Get Your Health Right" Hip-Hop Summits. We need "Get Your Health Right" lyrics, poetry, and images in rap and hip-hop video hits. Utilizing hip-hop as the means to raise public awareness about health has the potential to literally transform the world. We can and should begin to make a critical difference in this field of human endeavor and discipline.

It is a blessing to witness young health care professionals like Dr. Flowers, Dr. Davis and Dr. Joplin apply their skills and expertise to meet today's health challenges with the power of hip-hop culture and the latest advances in the provision of good health care. I AM HIP-HOP—I AM HEALTH represents a much needed synthesis and synergy between popular culture and the medical field. Health care is a fundamental basis for individual and community development. Health is a human right.

It is our hope that I AM HIP-HOP—I AM HEALTH will inspire the evolution of a global health and wellness movement led by advocates of hip-hop and health care professionals. This will be a participatory youth-led movement where everyone of every age and nation can participate.

In this book, the hot Tracks 1 through 9 are informative and the interludes from Russell Simmons, Missy Elliot, Too Poetic and Timbaland are all inspirational. School systems should use the book as well as we should make the text of these jewels readily available to students and youth everywhere.

I am reminded of when I had another blessed opportunity to work with that rising hip-hop star from the DipSet named Jim Jones on his latest album entitled, "HUSTLER'S POME: Product of My Environment." On Jim Jones' joint "Concrete Jungle," we together shouted out, "Yo, it definitely is a concrete jungle; and yet there is more to life than misery......... Life or death, you have to choose life." For too many young people today life is like a jungle of contradictions. But in life's circumstances you have to be willing to choose life over death when given a choice or an opportunity to improve your health.

Read I AM HIP-HOP—I AM HEALTH with passion and may your life be filled with wellness and empowerment. Let's spit truth to power. Let's reawaken the sleeping masses. Health care for all. Long live the spirit of the hip-hop health and wellness movement.

Dr. Benjamin F. Chavis, Jr.
New York City, June 2007

Intro
The Movement

I Am Hip-Hop, I Am Health is a movement that uses hip-hop music to bring health and wellness education to hip-hop communities the world over. This movement will promote "the cooler side" of health education and awareness, while affecting change and saving lives. I Am Hip-Hop, I Am Health promotes a healthier lifestyle so you do not lose the healthier self you were yesterday and the healthier self you might become tomorrow.

Health is truly the greatest wealth. Without your health, you will never be able to hold, take, keep or create anything. We believe that hip-hop and pursuit of good health can have a common goal of developing a national action plan to address today's primary health concerns. Our health concerns today will become future hip-hop generations' concerns tomorrow. The youth can be our future or our fate. Our intentions with this book are to highlight the major health disparities affecting our culture today. Our intentions are not to sow fear, but rather to empower and encourage hip-hop communities of today and tomorrow. I Am Hip-Hop, I Am Health is a collaboration between two forces; the hip-hop culture and the health care culture. One is a vehicle and the other is the message.

I Am Hip-Hop, I Am Health is a needed movement. It is a catalyst to organize, mobilize and advance into a healthier world. We don't expect everyone to agree with our views. In fact, we are sure that some readers will disagree with the idea of hip-hop being used as a vehicle to educate youth about health disparities. But to those of you thinking this way, we ask that you remain open to the cause and the movement.

Since first emerging in New York City in the 1970s, hip-hop music has given voice to persons in poverty. Now almost 40 years later, hip-hop has grown to encompass not just rapping, but also an entire lifestyle that incorporates diverse elements of race and ethnicity, technology, art, community, spirituality, health, wealth and education. In this book, we are going to share with you our experiences growing up with energy for hip-hop, out thoughts on hip-hop's potential global influence on health, and our passion for health education.

Hip-hop music has always been deemed the voice of the people, the ghetto newspaper, or, as Public Enemy front man Chuck D has said, "Rap is the black CNN." As has always been the case with Black music, hip-hop articulated something so universal and revelatory that everyone wanted to listen in. Hip-hop broke through doors barring access to the mainstream, exploding onto radio, television and records, all with racial and cultural implications.

Hip-hop began a movement through the streets, social classes, media outlets, classrooms, universities, boardrooms and hospitals. Those of us who grew up with hip-hop brought it with us wherever we went in order to stay connected to a recognizable culture. Particularly when we found ourselves outside our comfortable culture, hip-hop provided a means of familiarity in an unfamiliar world. As we became maturing students and burgeoning professionals, hip-hop would help us relax, provide a rhythm of security, and offer a rhyme to our reason. Hip-hop also lent a flavor that often was absent in mainstream American education and business.

THE CONNECTION

Drs. Davis, Flowers and Joplin grew up with hip-hop, have stayed connected to hip-hop as health care professionals, and have now merged hip-hop with health to create I Am Hip-Hop, I Am Health.

The collaboration of hip-hop and health can be compared to the mind-body connection. This is a connection implying that anything affecting the health of the mind will affect the body. And in turn; anything that affects the health of the body will also affect the mind. You cannot separate the body and mind from one another. A sound mind leads to a sound body and a sound body leads to a sound mind.

Hip-hop has arguably demonstrated an impact on the thinking, health and actions of its listeners. Today you have to be completely out of touch with American culture not to be aware of the impact hip-hop is having on daily life. In our schools, colleges and business offices you can find listeners plugged into mp3 players, satellite music players, radios and compact disc players listening to hip-hop. These music players cause direct connections or download to the brain, sending signals to the mind, which in turn direct emotion and then in turn the body's action.

Your health begins with your consciousness. As you become more aware of your health and health care needs, you will be building a greater connection to wellness. With health awareness and good health practices, you will establish the groundwork for freedom from pain and disease.

Persons are understood to be healthy when all their mind-body systems are in balance and working properly. Poor health is when mind-body systems become compromised and function out of balance. Unfortunately, good health is not that simple. Multiple domains of the human experience influence health. Being healthy encompasses four overlapping parameters: psychological, spiritual, physiological, and social. For instance, someone who is depressed might be experiencing feeling of hopelessness, low energy, low self-esteem, poor concentration or poor appetite. The reason might be a physiological condition (such as heart trouble), a social condition (such as losing a loved one), or a psychological condition (such as an overly self-critical nature). An imbalance in any of these areas will likely prevent an individual from obtaining optimal health.

Track 1

Dr. Gary Davis,
Is Hip-Hop &
Health

I can remember hearing my first rap song as if it were yesterday.

Ahh fly girls, clap your hands
Ahh fly guys, clap your hands
Well if you're feeling alright and you think you're on
Ah-somebody let me know
Well everybody in the place put a whistle in your face
Scream it out and say yooooo, hit it!

Yep, The Sugar Hill Gang with the "8th Wonder" was my first exposure to rap music and would not be my last. During my youth I adored everything that rap music had to offer: the style, the fashion, the language, and the dance. Everything about rap was vibrant and colorful to me. It was like a magnet pulling me into its fields, shaping my thoughts and behavior. Rap music was educating me about problems in our nation's communities. It was the voice of truth, spoken from the youth unedited, uncut, and raw.

I embraced as much as I could of the rap culture even while under the tight reign of my mother. Looking back, I can now understand my mother's concern. Yeah, I had my share of flavored Lees, name-brand jeans, and Adidas sneakers. That was hot back in the day, but I wore them sparingly around my mother, because the media depicted those styles associated with nothing but ruthless, violent, gun-toting predatory brothers robbing one another. My mother was just trying to protect me.

As I reached my teens, I made attempts to get involved in the growing trend of rap music. I was a part of a dance group called the Supreme Poppers for about two years. Then my interest changed to the turntables, but that was very short-lived. I never tried to rap, but I was always interested to see and hear emcees battling on the corner.

There was something that I was accelerating in privately. My mother had for years fed my growing interest in science.

As a teenager, I would imitate a physician with my stethoscope and reflex hammer. I can recall hours spent looking at all types of substances under my microscope. The stage was set and the future written. I became a Doctor of Chiropractic with a strong interest in nutrition, structure and posture as it relates to health and wellness.

But I still adored what is now called hip-hop. I had the same feelings about it as when I was a kid growing up in Baltimore. And just as I have grown and evolved, so has hip-hop. Hip-hop has influenced every facet of American culture. It has reshaped music, fashion and the entertainment industry. Hip hop is a worldwide phenomenon, touching all ages, cultures and continents. It has become one of the most trend-setting forces in America. It has even given its audience new hope, and it has influenced politics. Witness the political agendas of Rap to Vote (Russell Simmons) and Vote or Die (Sean 'Diddy' Combs) in the 2000 campaigns for voter registration. Now is the time for me to partner my two passions, hip-hop and health!

Dr. Gary L. Davis, Jr., is a Doctor of Chiropractic. He is also certified in Manipulation Under Anesthesia (MUA) at the Norma Vista Hospital of Houston, Texas, and at the California Academy for Manipulation Under Anesthesia. He received further training for Manipulation Under Anesthesia at the Arizona Surgical Hospital in Phoenix, Arizona. He is licensed by the Virginia Board of Medicine and currently owns his own practice in Falls Church, VA. Dr. Davis is passionately committed to educating at-risk persons on health care issues and providing them with information to make better decisions for preventing and managing disease

Track 2

Why, I Am
Hip-Hop,
I Am Health Movement

Since the early '80s, hip-hop music has served as a powerful voice and form of expression for young black audiences. It has evolved into a culture with its own language, style of dress and mindset. But despite its popularity and appeal, few health organizations, nutrition institutes and associations have used hip-hop's ability to speak to the needs and values of black youth.

This is probably a lost opportunity. Both the youth that buys listens and internalizes the music, as well as the emcees, deejays and producers who create the music share knowledge, appreciation and love of the hip-hop culture. Incorporating hip-hop culture is a great way to motivate youth to share messages and increase participation in healthy lifestyle changes. But to do that well, you have to be knowledgeable about the culture and open to it.

In recent years, hip-hop artists have started publicly denouncing the unhealthy lifestyles some of their counterparts have long embraced. They are pushing the benefits of holistic health in the black community, where high blood pressure and cholesterol are common problems. Indeed, unhealthy lifestyles are an epidemic in the black community and are at least partly to blame for such diseases as cancer, arthritis, asthma, obesity and diabetes. Nearly 75 percent of African Americans have at least one health condition that is directly related to their lifestyle. Through music, hip-hop artists have the ability to deliver that message to their listeners.

Hip-hop can help millions of today's youth and young adults. It can lead the way out of the systematic physical slavery of poor health and health disparities that is 'normal' in today's society. Young people want a new way, something identifiable to them and their culture. Hip-hop is giving millions of persons a purpose that hypocrites in the government, schools and churches have failed to provide.

The implementation and gradual development of improved health care in communities will enhance self-awareness, self-esteem, personal pride and productivity. Providing health care programming will stimulate health consciousness and interest, which in turn can spark organizational and economic growth. Once the seeds of opportunity and personal accountability have been sown, organizations will be more likely to invest in future health care development and organizational growth opportunities. As the spirit of positive health and successful community life expand, additional programming and health care distribution can be implemented to the benefit of organizations and hip-hop community members.

Interlude: Russell Simmons

I began yoga in the mid 1990s with a good friend in Los Angeles. I have faithfully made yoga a staple in my life. In the mornings, I do my meditation, and in the middle of the day, physical practice. My staff knows to keep my schedule free during mid-day; that is my yoga time, and it is very important to me.

Yoga is about clearing and quieting the mind through asana (positions) practice, as well as meditation. It's about clearing the mind of fluctuations so you can one day find your true self. Buddhists refer to this state as nirvana, the Yogis as samadhi or simply as the state of yoga. Practicing yoga helps me quiet my inner-self and revitalizes my soul. Yoga helps me manage and enjoy my lifestyle. It is a way for me to reach spiritual enlightenment and find purpose in all that I do.

Yoga has definitely helped relieve the pressures of the office. It decreases stress while increasing circulation and flexibility. It is good for the heart; and the breathing and postures are good for the lungs. Just five minutes doing a headstand, thereby reversing your blood flow, is great for your body. Sitting still and meditating is good for your mind. It has a psychosomatic affect on the body. Yoga has a spiritual benefit as well as a physical benefit.

Practicing yoga also means causing the least amount of harm possible to the planet and all sentient beings. This is why some yogis believe that to achieve total enlightenment, the state of yoga, or samadhi, you must become a vegetarian.

That is what led me to become a vegan. I believe in yoga, so I chose to eliminate all animal products from my diet. There are many variations of vegetarianism, but I am a total vegan. I have a strict plant-based diet with no animal byproducts at all. I don't consume any animal products or dairy.

Some people believe that vegetarianism is a new wave of medicine for the future, because plants have many benefits for the prevention of diseases. My life has changed since I became a vegan. I feel healthier. I have lost weight. And I have more energy.

In addition, being a vegetarian is also about the ultimate expression of non-violence. Yoga has some very important principles that can lead us.

Five steps to choosing an exercise program:

1. **Consult your doctor before starting any exercise program.**
2. **Know your physical limitations before starting.**
3. **Have a plan: It should include exercises and weight loss goals or health goals.**
4. **Use a personal trainer for motivation.**
5. **Follow all safety rules to prevent injury while working out.**

Track 3

Dr. Ross Flowers
Is Hip-Hop &
Health

I *said a hip-hop the hippie the hippie*
to the hip hip-hop, a you don't stop the rock it to the bang bang
boogie say up jumped the boogie to the rhythm of the boogie, the
beat now what you hear is not a test— I'm rappin to the beat and me,
the groove, and my friends are gonna try to move your feet see I am
wonder mike and I like to say hello to the black, to the white, the red,
and the brown, the purple and yellow"

I fell in love with hip-hop when I learned the words to the Sugar Hill Gangs' record "Rappers Delight." I remember spittin' my version of the lyrics and feelin' cool! Cool enough that I found the courage to rap out loud and flow to girls that I thought were cute. I would try and imitate the voices and what I thought the rappers looked liked rhyming. MTV, VH1, BET, and The Box weren't out yet. So, my imagination ran wild with what I thought hip-hop was all about. I'll never forget trying to beat box and rap, trying to sound like the Sugar Hill Gang, Fat Boys, The Furious Five, or Afrika Bambaataa.

One of my earliest memories of hip-hop was playing 12" record after record with my older brother Chris downstairs in our parents' house, bobbin' our heads and trying to imitate what we heard on wax. Man, we'd listen to records for hours trying to figure out what was being said and memorize the lyrics. Listening to hip-hop made me feel alive.

One of my funniest memories of early hip-hop happened after I thought I had memorized "Rappers Delight." I called a girl that I liked at the time, and started flowin' over the phone. I got to the part where the emcee said *"to the black to the white, red and the brown, the purple and yellow."* But I added and mixed up the order of the colors. The girl was buggin' out over the phone laughing and calling her older brother to the phone to listen to me mess up the lyrics. But, I was still flowin' and could care less what that girl and her brother thought. I still had her on the phone, right! So what if my lyrics didn't always coincide with the actual lyrics of the song. I was rhymin' and the beat of hip-hop was hypnotic. From the early days of the Sugar Hill Gang, Afrika Bambaataa, Stetsasonic, Kool Mo D, Run DMC, KRS-1 and Boogie Down Productions through Ice-T, LL Cool J, NWA, Big Daddy Kane, Eric B and Rakhim all the way through Biggie, 2-PAC, Nas, Jay-Z and today's recent artists, I knew right away that I was hooked to hip-hop!

In the same way that I had a jones for hip-hop, I had a passion for athletics. I started playing competitive sports at age four. I thrived on the challenge and the exhilaration of competition. Athletics has been an elusive internal itch that cannot be eradicated by success, failure, injury or retirement. For me, being athletic developed from running around the house with my grandfather to playing competitive youth sports, to high school and college intercollegiate athletics, through professional athletics, coaching, counseling and consulting with athletes, teams and universities.

The meaning of athletics changes as you grow. Early in life athletics is fun, challenging and developmental. As you grow, your specific interest rise and your skill levels build. Athletics becomes more than a hobby; it becomes a passion to fulfill. In the attempts to satisfy the itch of passion, athletics becomes a way of life, a way of developing your mind and body to live and be healthy in order to achieve athletic success. So, from the immature excitement and fun, through the developmental challenges and growth, to the knowledge and poise of satisfying a healthy mind and body, athletics is a way of life.

Things became very clear to me during college when my athletic aspirations were slammed by a career-threatening injury. It required surgery and at best could only offer an unknown prognosis for returning to competition. Mind and body health became my focus and passion. Understanding the connection between mind and body was crucial to my ability to manage surgery, rehabilitation, doubt and fear. I quickly realized that a strong, agile body was weak without a flexible mind and poised spirit.

When life involves conscious awareness of mind and body, and incorporates an infatuation with something you love, like hip-hop…. It's all love!

Through the eyes of health professionals who grew up in the hip-hop culture, we present what we have learned and experienced to be life-changing health care information and practices. We have also included notable experiences of those who have also been inspired by hip-hop and health.

I Am Hip-Hop! I Am Health!

Dr. Ross Flowers received his doctorate in counseling psychology with emphasis on performance enhancement from the University of Missouri-Kansas City. He is licensed as a psychologist in the state of California. Dr. Flowers is a psychologist and the director of sport psychology at the University of California, Davis. In addition to his work at the University of California, Davis, Dr. Flowers works with many celebrated USA, Olympic and international elite performers He is a member of the USA Track & Field Sport Psychology Executive Committee, and the Association of Applied Sport Psychology. Dr. Flowers has published in his areas of expertise, including; performance psychology, performance anxiety, and motivation.

Track 4

History and Influence of
Hip-Hop

There are four fundamental elements in hip-hop: Hip-hop dance (notably break dancing), urban inspired art (notably graffiti), deejaying and emceeing. Coinage of the term "hip-hop" is often credited to Keith Cowboy, a rapper in Grandmaster Flash & The Furious Five. Though LoveBug Starski, Keith Cowboy and DJ Hollywood used the term when the music was known as "Disco Rap," it is believed that Cowboy created the term while teasing a friend who had just joined the U.S. Army, by scat singing the words "hip/hop/hip/hop" in a way that mimicked the rhythmic cadence of marching soldiers. Cowboy later worked the "hip-hop" cadence into a part of his stage performance, which was quickly copied by other artists. An example is the Sugar Hill Gang in their opening of the single "Rapper's Delight." Afrika Bambaataa is credited with first using the term "hip-hop" to describe the culture that rap music belonged to, although an alternative theory is that the term was originally used—derisively—against the new type of music.

Old school hip-hop is the first hip-hop music to come out of the block parties of New York City in the 1970s and early 1980s. It began in the early 1970s with the advent of break beat deejaying, in which DJs extended the breaks of funk records, creating a more "danceable" sound. The early DJs at the parties began isolating the percussion breaks of hit songs—realizing that these were the most danceable and entertaining parts—and extending them, using an audio mixer and two records. At the time, this technique was common in Jamaica, and was known as dub music. It spread via the substantial Jamaican immigrant community in New York City, especially via the godfather of hip-hop, DJ Kool Herc. The use of extended percussion breaks led to the development of mixing and scratching techniques, and later to the popularization of remixes.

As hip-hop's popularity grew, performers began speaking ("rapping") in sync with the beats, and became known as emcees.

Teams of emcees sprang up throughout the country. Frequently, these were collaborations among former gang members, such among those of Afrika Bambaataa's Universal Zulu Nation (now a large international organization). The Herculoids and other early performers focused on introducing themselves and others in the audience (the origin of the still common practice of "shouting out" on hip-hop records). These early emcee teams often spoke for hours at a time, with some improvisation and a simple four-count beat, along with a basic chorus (for example, "one, two, three, y'all, to the beat, y'all") to allow the performer to gather his thoughts. Later, the emcees grew more varied in their vocal and rhythmic approach, incorporating brief rhymes, often with a sexual or scatological theme, in an effort at differentiating themselves and entertaining the audience. These early raps incorporated similar rhyming lyrics from African American culture (see roots of hip-hop music), such as the dozens.

During the early 1970s, b-boying—more popularly known as breaking—arose during block parties, as b-boys and b-girls got in front of the audience to dance in a distinctive, frenetic style. The style was documented for release to a world wide audience for the first time in the movie "Beat Street", though it could be argued that the movie "Flashdance" offered the first glimpse to a world wide audience. The style was also prominently featured a year earlier in both movies "Style Wars" and "Wildstyle", but one could argue these were not world wide releases.

Currently, as a cultural movement, hip-hop manages to get billed as both a positive and negative influence on young people, especially on Black and Latino youth. On one hand, there are African American activists, artists and entrepreneurs, such as Russell Simmons, who seek to build a progressive political movement among young hip-hop fans and who have had modest success with voter registration efforts. On the other hand, there's no shortage of critics who denounce the negative portrayals of Black people, especially women, in hip-hop lyrics and videos.

The study of the hip-hop generation fails to definitively answer the big question: Do rap music and other traits of the hip-hop culture influence teens or merely mirror the culture that teens have created? The answer is probably both. After more than two decades of hip-hop growth, today's scholars who grew up in the Old School (1970-1986) and Golden Age (1986-1993) of Hip-Hop may one day provide clear answers to questions of hip-hop's influence.

But let's assume a considerable influence. Then consider this: If young Black America is going to be a cultural trendsetter worldwide, why not use this to our advantage? Can you imagine what our influence could be if more groups like The Fugees or A Tribe Called Quest created music and lyrics to inspire a new wave in Pan-African thinking? If hip-hop is destined to rule youth culture around the world, wouldn't you rather it is a reign that will unite and empower Black people everywhere?

Interlude: Missy Elliot

"I still represent for overweight adults and kids but I am now painfully and personally aware of the health issues,"

Missy Elliott is hip-hop and she is health. Elliott explained that she was diagnosed with hypertension and that in her past had been seriously ill. Her condition was complicated by kidney stones and gallstones.

"I was too young to be dealing with that. Those are when you get older. You know grandmothers and grandfathers with stuff like that. High blood pressure, that's the silent killer. And that's like the biggest thing that runs through my family. Everybody in my family is on high-blood-pressure pills. And what's scariest is not knowing that your pressure is up. It's why they call it "the silent killer," 'cause you can end up dying from it. A lot of people have passed away from having high blood pressure and didn't know. One lady was telling me how she had a stroke from her pressure being high. She said she was in a classroom, teaching, and all of a sudden her whole right side went numb. I ain't trying to leave here, not this early."

Five Steps to Managing Hypertension:

1) Keep a record of your blood pressure and review it often with your doctor.
2) Monitor your weight and diet. Keep sweets to a minimum.
3) Participate in regular exercises (20 minutes physical activity daily or cardio workout 30 minutes three times a week).
4) Never self medicate. If on medication, take it as prescribed by your doctor.
5) Decrease your intake of salty food/snack.

Track 5

Health Disparities

Obesity

Diabetes Mellitus

Cardiovascular Disease

Cancer

Hypertension

HIV/AIDS

OBESITY

Aim for a Healthy Weight
- Determine your Body Mass Index (BMI).
- If you are overweight or obese, losing just 10% of your body weight can improve your health.
- If you need to lose weight, do so gradually—1/2 to 2 pounds a week.

Be Active
- Keep physically active to balance the calories you consume.
- Be physically active for at least 30 minutes (adults) or 60 minutes (children) on most days of the week.
- Limit TV time to less than two hours a day.

Eat Well
- Select sensible portion sizes.
- Follow the Dietary Guidelines for Americans shown at www.health.gov/dietaryguidelines.

What Weight Measure is Used?
- An expert panel, convened by the National Institutes of Health in 1998, recommended that Body Mass Index (BMI) be used to classify overweight and obesity.

Why is BMI Used?
- BMI correlates with risk of disease and death. For example, heart disease increases with increasing BMI in all population groups.
- Calculating BMI is simple, rapid, and inexpensive.
- BMI correlates well with total body fat for the majority of people.

Determining BMI
- BMI is a measure of weight in relation to height:

$$\frac{\text{weight (kg)}}{\text{height (m)2}} \quad \text{or} \quad \frac{\text{weight (pounds) x 703}}{\text{height (inches)2}}$$

- As an alternative to calculating BMI, tables to

determine BMI are commonly available at www.nhlbi.
nih.gov/guidelines/obesity/bmi_tbl.htm.

Classification of Overweight and Obesity by BMI

- In adults:
  {Healthy weight 18.5-24.9}
  {Overweight 25.0-29.9}
  {Obesity Class I 30.0-34.9}
- In children and adolescents aged 6 to 19 years, being
  overweight has been defined as a sex- and age-specific
  BMI at or above the 95th percentile, based on revised
  Centers for Disease Control and Prevention growth
  charts (shown on www.cdc.gov/growthcharts).

[BMI has some limitations. It can overestimate body fat in
persons who are very muscular, and it can underestimate body
fat in persons who have lost muscle mass, such as many elderly
persons. An actual diagnosis of overweight or obesity should be
made by a health professional.]

Health Consequences

- Overweight and obesity are associated with heart
  disease, certain types of cancer, Type 2 diabetes,
  stroke, arthritis, breathing problems and psychological
  disorders such as depression.
- Having a BMI in the overweight or obese range does
  not necessarily indicate that a person is unhealthy.
  Other risk factors, such as high blood pressure, high
  cholesterol, smoking, diabetes, and personal and
  family medical history are important to consider when
  assessing overall health.
- The higher a person's BMI is above 25, the greater
  their weight-related health risks.

DIABETES MELLITUS

Aim for a Decrease in Diabetes

In recent years, the Food and Drug Administration has taken steps that make it possible for people with diabetes to maintain better control of their disease. In the early 1990s, the agency, along with the U.S. Department of Agriculture, put in place food labeling regulations that, among other things, require labels of most packaged foods to provide nutrition information. Thus people with diabetes can now learn about the nutritional content of almost all the foods they eat.

Be Active

- Keep physically active to balance the calories you consume.
- Aim for a healthy weight.

Eat Well

- Let the Food Pyramid guide your food choices. (see www.FDA.gov)
- Choose a variety of grains daily, especially whole grains.
- Choose a variety of fruits and vegetables daily.
- Keep food safe to eat.

What Measure is Used?

Whatever method used, ADA recommends these general dietary guidelines for people with diabetes:
- Limit fat to 30 percent or less of daily calories.
- Limit saturated fat to 10 percent or less of daily calories.
- Limit protein to 10 to 20 percent of daily calories. For those with initial signs of diabetes-induced kidney disease, restrict protein to 10 percent of daily calories.
- Limit cholesterol to 300 milligrams or less daily.
- Consume about 20 to 35 grams of fiber daily.

Why These Guidelines are Used

ADA recommends a calorie reduction of 250 to 500

calories from what is normally eaten in a day. This should result in a weight loss of about 0.2 to 0.5 kilograms, or 1/2 to 1 pound a week. Calorie restriction, along with increased exercise, should help an overweight person achieve a weight loss of 5 to 10 kilograms, or 11 to 22 pounds, in about six months to a year. The weight loss, although moderate, can help improve diabetes control.

Determining Your Risk

Symptoms of untreated insulin-dependent diabetes include:

- Continuous need to urinate
- Excessive thirst
- Increased appetite
- Weakness
- Tiredness
- Urinary tract infections
- Recurrent skin infections, such as boils
- Vaginal yeast infections in women
- Blurred vision
- Tingling or numbness in hands or feet.

Classification of Diabetes Mellitus

Insulin-dependent, or Type 1, diabetes affects about five percent of all diabetics. It's also known as juvenile diabetes because it often occurs in people under 35 and commonly appears in children or adolescents.

Non-insulin-dependent, or Type 2, diabetes is the most common type. It results when the body produces insufficient insulin to meet the body's needs or when the cells of the body have become resistant to insulin's effect.

Health Consequences

By following the government's Dietary Guidelines for Americans, you can promote your health and reduce your risk for developing a chronic disease such as heart disease, certain types of cancer, diabetes, stroke and osteoporosis. The diseases listed above are the leading causes of death and disability among

Americans. Good diets can also reduce major risk factors for chronic diseases such as obesity, high blood pressure, and high blood cholesterol.

CARDIOVASCULAR DISEASE

Aim for Prevention
- Quit smoking!
- Commit to weight loss management.
- Engage in regular physical activity.
- Strictly manage chronic medical conditions.
- Risk-factor screening in adults should begin at age 20, with re-evaluation in five years or sooner if medical conditions warrant.

Be Active

People who are usually inactive can improve their health and well-being by becoming moderately and regularly active.

Physical activity need not be strenuous to achieve health benefits.

Greater health benefits can be achieved by increasing the amount (duration, frequency or intensity) of physical activity.

An example of moderate exercise is 30 minutes of walking; "regular" means most or all days of the week.

What Measure is Used?

Pooled or parallel analyses of epidemiologic data from existing studies to better describe the diverse factors [e.g., ethnicity, age and environment (local disease patterns, early exposures and economic transition)] that may affect the relation between anthropometry and health;

Measurements of changes over time in individuals or populations to add a dynamic (time-dependent) aspect to risk assessment;

In addition to assessments of the risk of traditional mortality and morbidity endpoints, assessments of the risk of other important outcomes related to quality of life (e.g., back pain) that also seem related to being overweight;

Examinations of the extent to which various simple anthropometric indicators are confounded by height and the resulting effect of misclassifying individuals as obese or non-obese;

Considerations of ethnic and racial differences when anthropometric measures are used to assess health status; and

Incorporation of various simple anthropometric indicators into current national and community health surveys.

Why These Guidelines are Used
- Reduces the risk of dying prematurely
- Reduces feelings of depression and anxiety
- Helps build and maintain healthy bones, muscles, and joints
- Helps older adults become stronger with stability
- Promotes psychological well-being

Risk Factors
- Cigarette smoking
- Hypertension
- Hypercholesterolemia
- Diabetes
- Age greater than 50
- Male gender
- Family history
- Physical inactivity
- Obesity
- Chronic Inflammation (elevated C-reactive protein level)

Classification of Cardiovascular Disease
- *Acute Myocardial Infarction*: Sometimes called heart attack.
- *Aneurysm*: A sac formed by the dilation of the wall of an artery, a vein or the heart; it is filled with fluid or clotted blood often forming a pulsating tumor.
- *Angina Pectoris*: A symptomatic manifestation of ischemic heart disease, describing a severe squeezing or pressure-like thoracic pain, brought on by exertion or stress.
- *Arteriosclerosis*: A group of diseases characterized by thickening and loss of elasticity of arterial walls.

CANCER

Aim for a Decrease in Cancer

There is strong scientific evidence that healthy dietary patterns in combination with regular physical activity are necessary to maintain the body's ability to prevent cancer.

What Measure is Used?

The probability of developing cancer is calculated by DevCan which is owned by NCI. The probability takes into account the average experiences of everyone. There is no account for individual behavior and factors.

Why These Guidelines are Used

Statistical method called age-adjustment to compare groups of people with different age compositions; This is important when examining cancer rates because cancer is generally a disease of older adults.

Determining Your Risk

Anyone stands the risk of developing Cancer. The risk of being diagnosed with cancer increases with age. Most cases are in adults, middle aged and older. Relative risk is measured by the relationship between the risk factors and the type of cancer.

Classification of Cancer

Cancer is normally classified in two forms:

- Malignant—this type is the most dangerous because of its ability to spread from one tissue type to another.
- Benign—this form is considered localized to one tissue. Though considered dangerous, it results in a lower mortality rate.

Health Consequences

Lack of physical activity can affect your body's predisposition to certain cancers such as in the colon and breast.

HYPERTENSION

Aim for a Decrease in Hypertension
Barriers to effective management of hypertension:
- Lack of awareness about consequences of hypertension
- Lack of access to consumer medical information
- Later diagnosis and greater burden of disease at diagnosis
- Living in a disadvantaged neighborhood Inadequate resources to support healthy lifestyle choices
- Dietary factors, particularly low potassium, high sodium, and high fat intake
- High incidence of overweight in children and obesity in adults
- Inadequate recreational activity
- Distrust of medical professionals
- Adverse medication effects (actual or anticipated)

Eat Well
You can help lower your blood pressure by eating foods that are part of a healthy diet. If you want to keep your blood pressure normal, the best diet is one that is low in salt, sugar and fat, and high in calcium, magnesium and potassium.

You should eat plenty of fruits, vegetables, nuts, whole grains, fish, poultry, and low-fat dairy products. You should limit red meat, sugar, fat, foods high in cholesterol, and alcohol. You also should try to stay at a healthy weight.

What Measure is Used?
When diagnosing hypertension your medical provider will use the following definitions suggested by the Seventh Joint National Committee (JNC 7).

Based upon the average of two or more properly measured readings at each of two or more visits after an initial screening, the following classifications are used:

Normal blood pressure: Systolic BP <120 mmHg and

Diastolic < 80 Pre-hypertension: Systolic BP 120-139 or Diastolic BP 80-89 Hypertension:
- Stage 1: Systolic BP 140-159 or Diastolic BP 90-99
- Stage 2: Systolic BP >160 or Diastolic BP >100

Patients with pre-hypertension (systolic 120-139 and/or diastolic 80-89), but without diabetes, chronic renal failure, or cardiovascular disease are treated with non-pharmacologic therapies such as weight reduction, sodium restriction, and avoidance of excess alcohol. They should also have their blood pressure measured every 12 months, because they are at significant risk of developing hypertension over time.

Why These Guidelines are Used

The USPSTF (United States Preventive Services Task Force) strongly recommends that clinicians screen adults aged 18 and older for high blood pressure. Please remember that regular cardiovascular exercise and a diet rich in fruits and vegetables while low in salt has been shown to help lower blood pressure. You should ask your medical provider to focus on the underlying genetic and social factors (such as environment, family history, and diet), that may play a role in you developing hypertension. By doing so, you and your healthcare provider can help reduce the burden of hypertension-related disease and death not only for African Americans, but for all Americans.

Determining Your Risk

Several factors have been associated with increasing one's risk of developing hypertension which include:

Family history (having a relative with high blood pressure)

Excessive alcohol use,

High salt intake,

Lack of exercise and

High sugar intake (which can increase one's risk for developing diabetes)

Classification of Hypertension
- White-coat hypertension (increased BP associated with stress of a visit to the doctor's office)

- Pseudo-hypertension (usually occurs in elderly individuals, with stiff, non-compressible vessels)
- Pre-hypertension
- Hypertension

Health Consequences

High blood pressure is often called the "silent killer" because you can feel just fine when you have it even though damage may be occurring throughout your body. Uncontrolled hypertension can cause strokes, which can lead to brain or neurological damage, heart failure, kidney disease and even death.

HIV/AIDS

Aim for a Decrease in HIV/AIDS
Patients infected with HIV face a complex array of medical, psychological, and social challenges. A strong provider-patient relationship, the assistance of a multidisciplinary care team, and frequent office visits are usually required to provide excellent care.

What Measure is Used?
It is very important to have a CD4 count and a viral load test done at your first doctor's visit. You should also have drug resistance testing. The results will provide a baseline measurement for future tests. CD4 cells, also called CD4+ T cells or CD4 lymphocytes, are a type of white blood cell that fights infection. HIV destroys CD4 cells, weakening your body's immune system. A CD4 count is the number of CD4 cells in a sample of blood.

Why These Guidelines are Used
The U.S. Department of Health and Human Services (HHS) provides HIV treatment guidelines to doctors and patients. These guidelines recommend that you take a combination of three or more medications in a regimen called Highly Active Antiretroviral Therapy (HAART). The guidelines list "preferred" HAART regimens. However, your regimen should be tailored to your needs.

Factors to consider in selecting a treatment regimen include:
- Drug resistance testing results
- Number of pills
- How often the pills must be taken
- If pills can be taken with or without food
- How the medications interact with one another
- Other medications you take
- Other diseases or conditions
- Pregnancy

Determining Your Risk

What risk-taking behaviors should be reviewed with patients? Patients infected with HIV who practice unsafe sex or inject drugs can infect others, be re-infected themselves with new HIV strains, or contract STDs, viral hepatitis or other infections. Abuse of alcohol or illicit drugs is directly harmful and may affect adherence to a complicated medical regimen. Accordingly, providers need a detailed understanding of their patients' risk-taking behaviors to guide patient education and counseling efforts and to assess the advisability of initiating antiretroviral treatment.

Classification of HIV/AIDS

There are other factors that influence sexual transmission of HIV, such as:

- Presence of other sexually transmitted diseases (STDs)
- Genital irritation
- Menstruation
- Lack of circumcision in men
- Taking birth control pills
- Hormone imbalances
- Vitamin and mineral deficiencies

Always use prevention strategies, such as condoms and safer sex practices.

Health Consequences

You may feel reluctant to talk with your health care provider about your high-risk behaviors. It can be difficult to change behaviors, even when you want to. However, it is important to be honest with your provider about risky activities. You and your provider can then discuss ways to minimize the risk of infecting others. If you are a woman, you and your doctor should discuss ways to prevent pregnancy. If you want to become pregnant, you and your doctor can talk about what you should do to prevent transmitting HIV to your baby.

Track 6

Dr. Che Joplin
Is Hip-Hop &
Health

*I'm the King of Rock, there is none higher, sucka emcee they call
me sire, to burn my Kingdom they must use fire, and I won't stop
rockin' til I retire..."*

These words are blasting through my radio as I get ready
for school. I am a little late and I know I will have to walk twice
as fast to get to class on time. I am new to the school and I
haven't made a lot of friends yet. I am spending most of my
time playing basketball on the school yard court at lunch. Half
the year is over and I am still learning the rules of high school
and finding my place among all the new faces and influences.

Hip-hop music has been the only constant in my life over
those past few years. I have been at a few different schools in a few
different states. Though I made some friends, we would move
before I really got comfortable where I was. Hip-hop music had
always made my transition to some of the new places easier to
bear. It has never been my passion to learn to emcee or deejay,
probably because I never felt I had any real talent with words.
I didn't think I could put words together like emcees could to
tell a story, but still it was a talent I appreciated. Emcees were
able to hold my complete attention for minutes at a time. I had
a passion to know the music, what was the most current song
on the block and who was bustin' the lyrics at that time. This
always gave me an "in" when it came to meeting new people.
The music was crossing boundaries and slowly becoming big. I
felt if I knew the music and what was new I would be accepted,
and I wanted to be down.

Looking back, while living as a teenager in California in the
mid-1980s, I could see that most boys my age were affiliated with
street gangs or had friends involved in gang activity, mimicking
gangster rap music as a way of fitting in. Ice T with DJ Evil E
with the track *"6 in the morning, police at my door..."* and the album
<u>*Straight Outta Compton*</u> by N.W.A. were the most influential at
the time. The music fueled my rebellion against authority and

allowed me to feel strong. This compelled me to doing things I knew were wrong, but I was willing to do them to fit in.

The music also made me see there are consequences for my actions and you have to be ready to pay the price for what you do. Sometimes that price is more than you may be willing to pay. I know I wasn't willing to live the lifestyle some of the artists had lived even if I found moments of courage through their words. I knew I wasn't that type of person and if they knew me they would say the same thing.

Many times I've thought my parents had no clue about my troubles. The idea comes through clearly with the track *"Parents Just Don't Understand"* by DJ Jazzy Jeff and The Fresh Prince, and in *"The Formula"* by The D.O.C. When I listened to these songs and I was in a critical life situation, I felt like they were reading my thoughts. Always being somewhat of an introvert and an introspective thinker, I was really able to identify with DJ Eric B and Rakhim when they released the album *Paid In Full* and the track *"I Aint No Joke."* I was able to identify with their style of hip-hop, which has been described as velvet-smooth flow and with the content of their complex internal rhymes, which displayed literate imagery. This provided a blueprint to how I could approach those adults that made the difference in my life. Most adults were able to see that even though my situation was not new to them, it was new to me and serious as well.

It's safe to say that I wasn't a ladies' man while in school even though I had a girlfriend or two. Some may consider me a late bloomer because I lost my virginity at age 16. "I need love" and "I can't live without my radio…" were very influential songs at this time in my life, not because of the lyrics, but because who rapped it. I used the messages from my favorite artist to help define my persona. L.L.Cool J was definitely someone I used as a pattern for my attitude. When talking to the ladies, I worked hard to make sure I exuded the same confidence that he displayed in his music. As a sophomore in high school, this was the only way I knew how to make my approach to girls. I figured if they loved LL Cool J they would at least like me. I was lacking two things, though, the confidence and the muscular body. I would do the things he said in the song, *"I'll give you a rose, pull out your chair before we eat..."* I learned two valuable lessons from that song. Most girls want that type of attention from boys they like, and a 15–year-old girl has no idea how to appreciate that type of attention.

Just like the hip-hop artist of the period, I was part of a crew. We found it difficult to hang out without being seen as a gang. We were all moving past high school and making plans to be lawyers, military people, engineers, and for me, an educator. The four of us were connected by the music. We would meet after school, have ciphers, and everyone would talk about who was the dopest emcee.

"Let's begin, what, where, why, or when will all be explained like instructions to a game See I'm not insane; in fact; I'm kind of rational when I be asking you, "Who is more dramatical?" This one or that one, the white one or the black one pick the punk, and I'll jump up to attack one KRS-One is just the guy to lead a crew right up to your face and dis you ..."

This was my introduction to the concept of Knowledge Reigns Supreme Over Nearly Everyone and the artistry of KRS-ONE. It was an understanding that I believed in my heart. Driven by the consciousness and political edge in hip-hop music, I felt the need to find my purpose in life, and that meant leaving the people I knew best.

Armed with the familiar sounds of groups such as B.D.P., Public Enemy, De La Soul, and A Tribe Called Quest, I eventually arrived in Virginia and continued to find confidence and purpose throughout my college years. During this time, hip-hop music inspired black pride, unity, and self-awareness. I used the diverse range of topics and Afro-centric messages in the music to inspire me to pursue my interest in science and health. It was my way of giving back and affecting the black communities in a positive way.

The changes in my choice of hip-hop music have come about as I have grown, matured and evolved. The music has developed, just as I have. I am more confident now in my leadership and in my ability to make decisions, and I am better at making choices when it comes to what the newer hip-hop emcees are saying and their effects. Getting from where I began to where I am now has been largely influenced by various songs, artists and passions to give back. I am a fan, a lover of the music and a child of hip-hop's marriage to the politicized, Afro-centric consciousness of a culture at its breaking point. I am hip-hop personified and what hip-hop can be. I know music has made an impact on my decisions and on the kind of work that I am doing now.

Dr. Che Joplin completed his studies at Virginia State University where he received his undergraduate degree in Biology Research. He went on to complete his Doctorate of Chiropractic degree at Palmer College of Chiropractic in 1999. He completed further training at the California Academy for Manipulation Under Anesthesia. Dr. Joplin is a participating member of the following non-profit organizations: H2H Communications and Upliftment Jamaica. He is licensed by the Virginia Board of Medicine and is currently in private practice in Falls Church, Virginia.

Track 7

What the Hip-Hop Industry Can Do

We are calling on leading hip-hop organizations, records companies/labels, artist, and health providers to organize and lead the, I Am Hip-Hop, I Am Health, campaign and foster health initiatives across cities and college campuses to increase awareness about the state of health in the hip-hop generation. The following workshops can be used as a guide for the promotion of health and hip-hop in our global communities.

WORKSHOP NAME: HIP-HOP, HEALTH & EDUCATION: USING HIP-HOP AS A TOOL FOR EFFECTIVE PREVENTION COMMUNICATION

1) A Public Health Spin to hip-hop: Have youth share a healthy meal or snack with a distinguished local hip-hop guest. This might be a DJ, hip-hop artist, graffiti artist, music producer, artist manager, record label executive, dancer, clothing designer or graphic artist.

2) What Role Can hip-hop Have in the Classroom? Provide a canvas (a wall, paper, t-shirts) for your youth to express their feelings on nutrition and activity. They can create logos, pictures, murals, or collages using paint, markers or magazine cutouts.

3) The Impact of Mentoring on the Hip-hop Generation: Create a mentoring program using hip-hop music as a connecting point.

WORKSHOP NAME: CREATING THE POLICY DOCUMENT: DOCUMENTING YOUTH PERSPECTIVES

1) Create "A New School Agenda on Health and Education for America's Youth" Policy Document. Talk with school boards and superintendents about health lunches and snacks.

2)   Why Is It Important for Youth to Understand? Create a pledge for youth to understand the importance of health and physical activity.

WORKSHOP NAME: CREATING THOUGHT-PROVOKING RAPS WITH HEALTH/ED MESSAGES

1)   Meditation/Prayer/Relaxation (teaching meditation and relaxation techniques)

2)   Entertainment Education: Is It A Successful Communication Strategy for Reaching Youth? (Innovative multimedia approaches to youth programming)

3)   The hip-hop In "Storytelling" (Allowing youth to create storytelling rhymes with positive and healthy messages)

4)   Hip-hop's Role in Educating and Entertaining Youth (hip-hop music is a form of expression youth can use to channel their thoughts and feelings on health and related topics. Use hip-hop music to inspire physical activity; play hip-hop music during programming, games, and activity)

WORKSHOP NAME: OBESITY, HYPERTENSION, CANCER, HIV/AIDS & DIABETES AMONG THE HIP-HOP GENERATION

1)   How Do We Use hip-hop as a Catalyst to Reverse the Trends?

WORKSHOP NAME: PRIMARY HEALTH CARE & HIP-HOP: IS THERE A RELATIONSHIP?

1)   Communicating alternatives to youth about obesity, hypertension, cancer, HIV/AIDS and diabetes

2)   How to Reach The Hip-hop Generation With Key Information About Primary Health Care.

3)   Psychological Trauma In hip-hop—Ways to Recognize & Deal With It

Track 8

What Individuals Can Do

I Am Hip-Hop, I Am Health addresses health and wellness issues through strategic national and community initiatives and partnerships with private and public institutions. It is a health movement that takes a broad view of health, wellness and prevention. The movement is committed to helping build healthy and resilient lifestyles. Community residents of all economic levels are able to achieve their maximum health and wellness potential. The movement includes:

- Early intervention, wellness, health promotion, and health maintenance programs as the primary approach for solving health problems in the country.
- Encouragement of national and local corporations, organizations and educational facilities to be actively involved in the pursuit of community health and wellness.
- Improved data collection and research to help underserved communities understand health status and risk factors.
- Work to secure healthier communities through summits, media, and lectures while encouraging youth to take responsibility for their health.
- Promotion of daily activities for children, teens, adults and seniors.
- Promotion of healthy eating habits.
- Education on the major health disparities, plus ways to prevent and treat them.
- Holding our elected officials responsible for ensuring access to adequate healthcare, treatment and wellness options.

Screening Test

Having an agenda is important. For more practical

prevention when it comes to your health and well-being, the checklist below will empower you to take charge of your health.

Checklist for Men

The following recommendations are based on scientific evidence about screening tests you should have. Take this checklist with you to your doctor's appointment to use as a helpful reminder when you are scheduled to have any of these tests done.

- Cholesterol Checks: Have your cholesterol checked at least every 5 years, starting at age 35. If you smoke, have diabetes, or if heart disease runs in your family, start having your cholesterol checked at age 20.
- Blood Pressure: Have your blood pressure checked at least every 2 years.
- Colorectal Cancer Tests: Begin regular screening for colorectal cancer at age 50. Your doctor can help you decide which test is right for you. How often you need to be tested will depend on which test you have.
- Diabetes Tests: Have a test to screen for diabetes if you have high blood pressure or high cholesterol.
- Depression: If you've felt "down," sad or hopeless, and have felt little interest or pleasure in doing things for two weeks straight, talk to your doctor about whether he or she can screen you for depression.
- Sexually Transmitted Diseases: Talk to your doctor to see whether you should be screened for sexually transmitted diseases, such as HIV.
- Prostate Cancer Screening: If you are considering having a prostate-specific antigen (PSA) test or digital rectal examination (DRE), talk to your doctor about the possible benefits and harms.
- Aspirin: Talk to your doctor about taking aspirin to prevent heart disease if you are older than 40, or if

you are younger than 40 and have high blood pressure, high cholesterol, diabetes, or if you smoke.

- Immunizations: Stay up-to-date with your immunizations.

Checklist for Women

The following recommendations are based on scientific evidence about screening tests you should have. Take this checklist with you to your doctor's appointment to use as a helpful reminder when you are scheduled to have any of these tests done.

- Mammograms: Have a mammogram every 1 to 2 years starting at age 40.
- Pap Smears: Have a Pap smear every 1 to 3 years if you have been sexually active or are older than 21.
- Cholesterol Checks: Have your cholesterol checked regularly starting at age 45. If you smoke, have diabetes, or if heart disease runs in your family, start having your cholesterol checked at age 20.
- Blood Pressure: Have your blood pressure checked at least every 2 years.
- Colorectal Cancer Tests: Have a test for colorectal cancer starting at age 50. Your doctor can help you decide which test is right for you.
- Diabetes Tests: Have a test to screen for diabetes if you have high blood pressure or high cholesterol.
- Depression: If you've felt "down," sad or hopeless, and have felt little interest or pleasure in doing things for two weeks straight, talk to your doctor about whether he or she can screen you for depression.
- Osteoporosis Tests: Have a bone density test at age 65 to screen for osteoporosis (thinning of the bones). If you are between the ages of 60 and 64 and weigh 154 pounds or less, talk to your doctor about whether you should be tested.
- Chlamydia Tests and Tests for Other Sexually Transmitted Diseases: If you under 26 and sexually active you should be tested for Chlamydia and

Human Papilloma Virus (HPV) or any other sexually transmitted disease. If you are older than 25, talk to your doctor to see whether you should be tested for Chlamydia and HPV or any other sexually transmitted disease.

- Aspirin: Talk to your doctor about taking aspirin to prevent heart disease if you are older than 45 and have high blood pressure, high cholesterol, diabetes, or if you are a smoker.
- Immunizations: Stay up-to-date with your immunizations.

What Else Can You Do To Stay Healthy?

Don't Smoke! But if you do smoke, talk to your doctor about quitting. You can take medicine and get counseling to help you quit. Make a plan and set a quit date. Tell your family, friends, and co-workers you are quitting. Ask for their support. If you are pregnant and smoke, quitting now will help you and your baby.

Eat a Healthy Diet! Eat a variety of foods, including fruit, vegetables, animal or vegetable protein (such as meat, fish, chicken, eggs, beans, lentils, tofu or tempeh) and grains (such as rice). Limit the amount of saturated fat you eat.

Be Physically Active! Walk, dance, ride a bike, rake leaves, or do any other physical activity you enjoy. Start small and work up to a total of 20 to 30 minutes of activity most days of the week.

Stay at a Healthy Weight! Balance the number of calories you eat with the number you burn off by your activities. Remember to watch portion sizes. Talk to your doctor if you have questions about what or how much to eat.

Drink Alcohol Only in Moderation! If you drink alcohol, one drink a day is safe for women, unless you are pregnant. If you are pregnant, you should avoid alcohol. Researchers don't know how much alcohol will harm a fetus. It is best not to drink any alcohol while you are pregnant. A standard drink is one 12-

ounce bottle of beer or wine cooler, one 5-ounce glass of wine, or 1.5 ounces of 80-proof distilled spirits.

Interlude: Too Poetic

Too Poetic (born Anthony Ian Berkeley, 1966, in Trinidad; died July 15, 2001 in California) was a rapper and producer from the horror core rap band Gravediggaz. Anthony collapsed in his home studio with stomach pains and was subsequently diagnosed with colon cancer. Given only four months to live, Poetic nonetheless kept up the struggle against cancer despite his initial refusal of chemotherapy in favor of a diet of herbs and fresh juice. Poetic began the treatment, however, after the cancer metastasized from his colon to his lungs. Financial support came from both fans and other artists, including the unexpected likes of Warren G.

During this period, Poetic collaborated with The Prodigy's Maxim Reality and Last Emperor under the name of Tony Titanium (given to him by Frukwan because titanium metal was "as hard as Poetic's will to live," and as a reference to the titanium valve in his chest through which he received chemotherapy). He also collaborated with them under his original name Too Poetic, as well as continuing work on the third Gravediggaz album. The subsequent release, Nightmare in A-Minor, was the darkest work the group had done. It makes many references to Poetic's cancer, perhaps most notably on the track "Burn Baby Burn" and on the Last Emperor's track "One Life," which extensively details his brutal battle with cancer.

SIX steps to early Cancer signs and prevention:

1) **Learn self-examinations techniques from your doctor to increase early detection.**
2) **Have annual colorectal screening and breast examinations.**
3) **Look for signs and symptoms that are new or unusual (blood in your stool or urine).**
4) **Monitor your body's response to cancer precursors such as smoking, processed sweeteners and high fat diets.**
5) **Talk to your doctor openly about your health.**
6) **Check family history.**

Track 9

What Can Leaders and Elected Officials Do?

The study of hip-hop has exploded on college and university campuses. This increase in critical analysis and dialogue on hip-hop along with the growth of political hip-hop organizations is fundamental to securing hip-hop's participation and contribution to healthcare and its ability to influence healthcare policy.

The future of hip-hop's political activism is no easy path. Socially and politically aware artists, spokespersons and organizers challenge the characteristics described in the subgenre, namely hypersexualization and materialism. The primary challenge of hip-hop is transforming its listeners from displaying symptoms of oppression to becoming agents of progressive change. Hip-hop media, academia, artists and entertainers can develop a critical role in the formation of health care agenda and policy.

Exacerbated by the complications associated with heart disease, diabetes and cancer, older voters are dying. Young people influenced by hip-hop are reaching the age where they are eligible to vote and are steadily becoming an electoral voice. The point of the I Am Hip-Hop, I Am Health movement is to develop socially conscious health change. It should be noted that a true health agenda can not solely be built on a social movement. It requires a critical mass of people to exercise an impulse to the health crisis. The worldwide health care agenda of the I Am Hip-Hop, I Am Health movement cannot be exclusive to the black communities just as hip-hop cannot survive as a movement on its own. For our global communities to make a real contribution to the larger healthcare crisis, they should use hip-hop to create internal political goals and use the I Am Hip-Hop, I Am Health movement as a possible vehicle.

There are steps we can take to show that we are ready for a change. Taking responsibility for our health is a two-way street that also requires changes from a legislatures and governments.

- Solidify, improve and expand the community health and wellness infrastructure
- Undertake proactive initiatives including older adult and child/adolescent health and wellness programs
- Increase access to health care for at-risk populations
- Respond to the needs of community organizations and agencies that are addressing health and wellness issues
- Harness information technology (Computer, Mass Media, Telecommunications) to ensure that community residents have accurate and relevant information as well as other support that is pertinent to health and wellness improvement
- Develop, implement and maintain an active capacity-building program aligned with foundation health and wellness priorities and responsive to community needs
- Expand the capacity of citizens and local communities to understand health and wellness issues, assess problems, set priorities and devise effective strategies for prevention campaigns
- Enlist the active involvement of governmental, community and organizational leaders in building the country's health and wellness infrastructure

- Create overlapping formal and informal networks dedicated to health and wellness provisions

- Support the public health sector (local, state, university) through selected partnerships, initiatives and targeted funding
- Strengthen other systems and sectors that affect community health and wellness

Outro: Timbaland

There is one goal Timbaland has not yet achieved. He wants to be buck. Since this past November, Timbaland has embarked on an extensive weight-loss program that has helped him drop dramatically from a bloated 331 pounds to, as of this writing, a husky 222 pounds. Concurrently he is incorporating a protein-rich diet into a training regimen geared to turn body fat into thick, protruding muscles.

"I don't want to be lean and cut. I want to be buck," says Timbaland during an otherwise quiet evening at his mansion. *"I just like that look. When you see horses, or animals, like you see a monkey or a gorilla, like, they cut. It's a freaky look. When you keep working out, you get to be almost like an animal,"* he continues. *"I like the veins popping out. I love all that."*

Timbaland's journey to physical nirvana began late last October. At the time Timbaland was an overworked and overweight, albeit mega-successful, record producer. He ate sporadically, worked long hours, didn't exercise, and didn't maintain a healthy diet. When he did eat, he consumed food in large portions. Eventually his obesity hastened the onset of health and medical problems such as sugar diabetes, high blood pressure, high cholesterol, and dry scalp. *"They say that when you're overweight, everything changes,"* says Timbaland. *"In pictures you look older. You looked stressed. Weight does something to your skin; it makes you look crazy."*

Now, thanks to losing more than 100 pounds in less than six months, Timbaland is no longer afflicted by his former ailments. Radically transforming himself from a fast-food-nation casualty to a Mr. Universe-in-Training has profoundly affected him. *"I'm trying to talk to the youth, I never really saw it. Your outer being is who you are as a person. People say no, but your outside affects who you are inside."*

Five steps to managing your weight:

1) **Portion control is key. Remember that a "serving" is one cup (about the size of your fist).**
2) **Twenty minutes of physical activity daily is crucial. Start or join an exercise club at work or in your community.**
3) **Make sure your diet is balanced. A proper amount of protein and complex carbohydrates will fuel your body and not leave you hungry.**
4) **Add healthy snacks between meals to beat that afternoon decrease in energy.**
5) **Drink plenty of water, eight glasses of water daily.**

Credits: Endnotes

Www.miaminewtimes.com/issues/2005-04-07/news/feature.
html—35k—Jan 22, 2007

Www.idealog.us/2004/06/index.html—178k—Jan 23, 2007

Www.netweed.com/lyricalswords/2006_05_21_lyricalswords_
archive.html—60k -

Www.hiphopmusic.com/archives/002069.html—41k

Www.postgradmed.com/issues/2002/10_02/douglas_intro.
htm—10k -

Www.blackhealthcare.com/BHC/Hypertension/Description.
asp—23k -

Www.postgradmed.com/issues/2002/10_02/bakris3.htm—39k -

If hip-hop ruled the world—the gangsta music and lifestyle
as presented globally by the current music of US Black youth
culture should be changed to generate unity and empowerment—
Column—Brief Article Essence, March 1998 by Aisha Finch

Dr. Beatrice Bridglall, the assistant director of the Institute for
Urban and Minority Education at Columbia University.

Decoding hip-hop's cultural impact: scholars are poised to take
a close look at the influence of hip-hop on the social identity,
values of today's youth Black Issues in Higher Education, April
22, 2004 by Ronald Roach

Wikipedia® is a registered trademark of the Wikimedia
Foundation, Inc. http://en.wikipedia.org/wiki/Hip_hop

http://www.allhiphop.com/hiphopnews/?ID=5489By   Bhavna
Malkani Date: 3/23/2006 10:50 am

Diabetes.niddk.nih.gov/dm/pubs/africanamerican/—15k -

Www.blackhealthcare.com/BHC/Diabetes/Description.asp—
31k -

Www.blackwomenshealth.com/diabetes.htm—41k

Www.americanheart.org/presenter.jhtml?identifier=3010188—35k -

Www.nlm.nih.gov/medlineplus/heartdiseases.html—65k

Diabetes.niddk.nih.gov/dm/pubs/statistics/index.htm—42k

Www.zmag.org/content/showarticle.cfm?ItemID=10365—16k

American Cancer Society. Cancer facts and figures for African Americans 2000-2001. Atlanta, GA: American Cancer Society; 2000.

Ries LAG, Eisner MP, Kossary CL, Hankey BF, Miller BA, Edwards BK, editors. SEER cancer statistics review, 1973-1997. Bethesda, MD: National Cancer Institute; 2000

Centers for Disease Control and Prevention. Youth risk behavior surveillance—1999. MMWR Morb Mortal Wkly Rep 2000; 49:1-96.

Institute of Medicine. Haynes MA, Smedley BD, editors. The unequal burden of cancer. An assessment of NIH research and programs for ethnic minorities and the medically underserved. Washington, DC: National Academy Press; 1999

Ross, H. Lifting the unequal burden of cancer on minorities and the underserved. Office of Minority Health. US Department of Health and Human Services. Closing The Gap; 2000 August issue.

Centers for Disease Control and Prevention. Cigarette smoking among adults-United States, 1995. MMWR Morb Mortal Wkly Rep 1997; 46(51): 1217-20.

US Department of Health and Human Services. Healthy People 2010. Washington, DC: US Government Printing Office; 2000.

US Department of Health and Human Services. Physical activity and health: a report of the Surgeon General. Atlanta, GA: Centers for Disease Control and Prevention, National Center for Chronic Disease Prevention and Health Promotion; 1996.

Anderson LM, May DS. Has the use of cervical, breast, and colorectal cancer screening increased in the United States? Am J Public Health 1995; 85(6):840-2.

Davis, G. L. Editor of H2H magazine, interview with Russell Simmons copyright 2004 H2H communications, 1st edition, 1st vol.

All artist lyrics were quoted from www. Lyrics.com

Ries LAG, Harkins D, Krapcho M, Mariotto A, Miller BA, Feuer EJ, Clegg L, Eisner MP, Horner MJ, Howlader N, Hayat M, Hankey BF, Edwards BK (eds). SEER Cancer Statistics Review, 1975-2003, National Cancer Institute. Bethesda, MD, http://seer.cancer.gov/csr/1975_2003/, based on November 2005 SEER data submission, posted to the SEER web site, 2006.

Www.nlm.nih.gov/medlineplus/aids.html — 71k— Feb 3, 2007 - Www.niddk.nih.gov/health/nutrit/nutrit.htm — 12k

www.ingramcontent.com/pod-product-compliance
Lightning Source LLC
Chambersburg PA
CBHW050556280326
41933CB00011B/1872

* 9 7 8 1 4 2 4 3 3 7 4 1 5 *